The whole anti-inflammatory diet for beginners

A free guide and simple meal plan with easy recipes to heal the immune system and optimize a healthy living

Dorothy Cook

William Lulu

Table of contents:

In a world filled with dietary trends and health fads, it's refreshing to come across a guide that not only promises a path to wellness but also grounds itself in scientific understanding and practicality. "The Anti-Inflammatory Diet for Beginners" is a beacon of clarity in the often confusing landscape of nutrition.

As we navigate our daily lives, the impact of our food choices on our well-being cannot be overstated. Inflammation, a silent culprit behind many health issues, is a key player in the intricate dance of our bodies. This book serves as a thoughtful and accessible companion, demystifying the concept of an anti-inflammatory diet and providing a roadmap for those eager to embark on a journey toward better health.

The author seamlessly weaves together evidence-based information with actionable steps, making this guide suitable for both newcomers to the world of nutrition and those well-versed in its complexities. From understanding the science behind inflammation to practical meal plans and delicious recipes, this book is a holistic approach to wellness.

What sets this guide apart is its emphasis on simplicity and sustainability. The anti-inflammatory lifestyle need not be a daunting or restrictive journey, and this book masterfully guides you through the process of making informed choices without sacrificing the joy of eating.

Whether you're seeking relief from chronic conditions or simply aiming for a more vibrant life, "The Anti-Inflammatory Diet for Beginners" is a reliable compass. It not only empowers you to take control of your health but also invites you to savor the journey towards a balanced and inflammation-free life.

Here's to your health and the wisdom shared within these pages.

Chapter 1.

Introduction to Anti-Inflammatory Diet

In recent years, there has been a growing interest in the relationship between diet and inflammation, leading to the emergence of the anti-inflammatory diet as a popular approach to promoting overall health and well-being. This dietary strategy revolves around consuming foods that possess anti-inflammatory properties, aiming to reduce chronic inflammation in the body, which is linked to various health issues such as heart disease, diabetes, and arthritis.

Understanding Inflammation:

Inflammation is a natural response of the body to injury or infection. However, when inflammation becomes chronic, it can contribute to the development and progression of several chronic diseases. The anti-inflammatory diet focuses on mitigating this chronic inflammation by emphasizing the consumption of foods that are believed to have anti-inflammatory effects.

Core Principles of the Anti-Inflammatory Diet:

1. Whole Foods:

The foundation of the anti-inflammatory diet is built on whole, nutrient-dense foods. This includes fruits, vegetables, whole grains, lean proteins, and healthy fats. These foods are rich in vitamins, minerals, antioxidants, and other bioactive compounds that can help combat inflammation.

2. Omega-3 Fatty Acids:

Foods high in omega-3 fatty acids, such as fatty fish (salmon, mackerel, and sardines), flaxseeds, and walnuts, are integral to an anti-inflammatory diet. Omega-3s have been shown to have anti-inflammatory properties, playing a crucial role in reducing inflammation in the body.

3. Antioxidant-Rich Foods:

Antioxidants are potent compounds that neutralize free radicals, which contribute to inflammation. Berries, dark leafy greens, nuts, and colorful vegetables are excellent sources of antioxidants and are staples in the anti-inflammatory diet.

4. Spices and Herbs:

Turmeric, ginger, garlic, and cinnamon are examples of spices and herbs that are frequently included in the anti-inflammatory diet. These ingredients contain bioactive compounds with anti-inflammatory and antioxidant properties.

5. Probiotics and Fermented Foods:

Gut health is closely linked to inflammation, and the anti-inflammatory diet often incorporates probiotics found in yogurt, kefir, and fermented foods like sauerkraut and kimchi. These promote a healthy balance of gut bacteria, positively influencing inflammation.

Foods to Limit or Avoid:

1. Processed and Sugary Foods:

Highly processed foods and those

high in added sugars are known to promote inflammation. The anti-inflammatory diet encourages the reduction or elimination of these items to maintain overall health.

2. Refined Carbohydrates:

Foods with refined carbohydrates, such as white bread and sugary cereals, can contribute to inflammation. Choosing whole grains instead supports the anti-inflammatory principles.

3. Trans Fats:

Trans fats, often found in fried and commercially baked goods, are linked to inflammation and should be minimized in an anti-inflammatory diet.

Potential Benefits:

Adopting an anti-inflammatory diet is associated with various health benefits, including reduced risk of chronic diseases, improved heart health, better weight management, and enhanced overall well-being. However, it's essential to note that individual responses to dietary changes may vary, and consulting with a healthcare professional or a registered dietitian is recommended before making significant adjustments to one's diet.

In conclusion, the anti-inflammatory diet is a holistic approach to nourishing the body with foods that support overall health and combat chronic inflammation. By prioritizing whole, nutrient-dense foods and avoiding pro-inflammatory choices, individuals may experience improved well-being and a reduced

risk of various health conditions.

Chapter 2.

Understanding Inflammation and its Effects on Health

Inflammation is a natural and crucial part of the body's immune response, playing a pivotal role in defending against harmful invaders, such as bacteria, viruses, and injuries. However, when inflammation becomes chronic or uncontrolled, it can have detrimental effects on health.

At its core, inflammation is the body's complex biological response to harmful stimuli. It involves a cascade of events orchestrated by the immune system, with various cells and signaling molecules working together to eliminate the threat and promote tissue repair. Acute inflammation is a short-lived and localized response that aims to eradicate the cause of cell injury, clear out damaged cells, and initiate tissue repair.

On the other hand, chronic inflammation is a persistent and prolonged state of inflammation that can arise from various factors, including persistent infections, autoimmune disorders, or exposure to environmental irritants. Unlike acute inflammation, which is a protective and temporary response, chronic inflammation can contribute to the development of various diseases.

One of the primary concerns with chronic inflammation is its link to various health conditions, including cardiovascular diseases, diabetes, neurodegenerative disorders, and certain cancers. Inflammation can lead to damage and dysfunction of tissues and organs over time, contributing to the progression of these chronic diseases.

The role of inflammation in cardiovascular health is particularly noteworthy. Chronic inflammation can contribute to the formation of atherosclerosis, a condition characterized by the buildup of fatty deposits in the arteries. This process can lead to the narrowing and hardening of the arteries, increasing the risk of heart attacks and strokes.

Inflammation's impact on metabolic health is also significant, as it has been implicated in the development of insulin resistance and type 2 diabetes. The inflammatory response can interfere with the normal functioning of insulin, a hormone crucial for regulating blood sugar levels, leading to elevated glucose levels and insulin resistance.

In the realm of neurodegenerative disorders, chronic inflammation is thought to play a role in the progression of conditions like Alzheimer's disease and Parkinson's disease. Inflammation can contribute to the destruction of nerve cells and the formation of abnormal protein aggregates, characteristic features of these debilitating conditions.

Moreover, there is emerging evidence suggesting that chronic inflammation may influence cancer development. Inflammatory processes within the body can create an environment conducive to the growth and survival of cancer cells. Inflammatory cells and signaling molecules can promote angiogenesis (the formation of new blood vessels) and contribute to the invasion and metastasis of cancer cells.

Understanding inflammation and its effects on health is crucial for developing strategies to manage and prevent chronic inflammatory conditions. Lifestyle factors, such as diet, exercise, and stress management, can significantly influence the inflammatory response. Adopting an anti-inflammatory diet rich in fruits, vegetables, and omega-3 fatty acids, along with maintaining a healthy weight and engaging in regular physical activity, can help mitigate chronic inflammation and support overall health.

In conclusion, while inflammation is a vital and protective aspect of the body's immune system, its dysregulation and persistence can lead to a range of health problems. Recognizing the link between chronic inflammation and various diseases underscores the importance of adopting a holistic approach to health that addresses lifestyle factors and promotes a balanced immune response.

Chapter 3.

Benefits of an Anti-Inflammatory Diet

An anti-inflammatory diet has gained increasing attention in recent years for its potential health benefits. This dietary approach focuses on consuming foods that help reduce inflammation in the body, which is linked to various chronic conditions. Here are several key benefits associated with adopting an anti-inflammatory diet:

1. Reduced Risk of Chronic Diseases:

Chronic inflammation is believed

to contribute to the development of various diseases, including heart disease, diabetes, and certain cancers. An anti-inflammatory diet, rich in fruits, vegetables, and whole grains, has been shown to lower the risk of these conditions.

2. Joint Health:

Inflammation plays a significant role in joint pain and conditions like arthritis. By following an anti-inflammatory diet, individuals may experience relief from joint pain and stiffness, improving overall joint health and mobility.

3. Weight Management:

- Obesity is often associated with chronic inflammation. An anti-inflammatory diet encourages the consumption of nutrient-dense foods, which can contribute to weight management and, in turn, reduce inflammation.

4. Improved Gut Health:

The gut microbiome has a profound impact on the immune system and inflammation. An anti-inflammatory diet, with its emphasis on fiber-rich foods and probiotics, promotes a healthy balance of gut bacteria, contributing to improved digestion and reduced inflammation.

5. Heart Health:

Chronic inflammation is a risk factor for cardiovascular diseases. Adopting an anti-inflammatory diet that includes heart-healthy fats, such as those found in olive oil and fatty fish, can positively impact cholesterol levels and lower the risk of heart-related issues.

6. Balanced Blood Sugar Levels:

-Chronic inflammation is linked to insulin resistance and diabetes. An anti-inflammatory diet that includes whole, unprocessed foods can help regulate blood sugar levels and reduce the risk of developing type 2 diabetes.

7. Enhanced Brain Health:

Inflammation has been implicated in neurodegenerative diseases such as Alzheimer's and Parkinson's. Consuming anti-inflammatory foods, rich in antioxidants and omega-3 fatty acids, may contribute to improved cognitive function and overall brain health.

8. Healthy Aging:

Chronic inflammation is associated with accelerated aging. An anti-inflammatory diet can potentially slow down the aging process by reducing oxidative stress and inflammation, leading to healthier aging and improved longevity.

9. Better Mood and Mental Health:

There is evidence linking

inflammation to mental health conditions like depression. Following an anti-inflammatory diet may positively impact mood and mental well-being, providing an additional avenue for mental health support.

10. Increased Energy and Vitality:

By eliminating or reducing inflammatory foods, individuals may experience increased energy levels and overall vitality. This can contribute to a more active and fulfilling lifestyle.

In conclusion, adopting an anti-inflammatory diet is a holistic approach to promoting overall health and well-being. While it's not a cure-all, the evidence suggests that incorporating anti-inflammatory principles into one's diet can have a positive impact on various aspects of health, from reducing the risk of chronic diseases to improving joint function and mental well-being. As with any dietary changes, it's essential to consult with a healthcare professional or a registered dietitian to ensure that the chosen diet meets individual nutritional needs.

Chapter 4.

Essential Nutrients and Foods for Fighting Inflammation

Inflammation is a natural immune response that helps the body fight off harmful invaders and promotes healing. However, chronic inflammation can contribute to various health issues, including heart disease, diabetes, and autoimmune disorders. Fortunately, adopting a diet rich in essential nutrients can play a crucial role in reducing inflammation and promoting overall well-being.

Omega-3 Fatty Acids

Omega-3 fatty acids are renowned for their anti-inflammatory properties. These essential fats are found in fatty fish like salmon, mackerel, and sardines. Incorporating these fish into your diet can provide eicosapentaenoic acid (EPA) and docosahexaenoic acid (DHA), which have been shown to suppress inflammation. Additionally, plant-based sources such as chia seeds, flaxseeds, and walnuts contain alpha-linolenic acid

(ALA), a precursor to EPA and DHA.

Antioxidants

A diet rich in antioxidants can help combat oxidative stress, a key contributor to inflammation. Colorful fruits and vegetables such as berries, cherries, spinach, and kale are packed with antioxidants like vitamins C and E, beta-carotene, and flavonoids. These compounds neutralize free radicals and reduce inflammation, supporting overall health.

Turmeric and Curcumin

Turmeric, a spice commonly used in Indian cuisine, contains curcumin, a powerful anti-inflammatory compound. Studies have suggested that curcumin can help modulate inflammatory pathways in the body. Adding turmeric to dishes or consuming curcumin supplements may contribute to reducing inflammation and alleviating symptoms associated with inflammatory conditions.

Ginger

Ginger has been used for centuries

for its medicinal properties, including anti-inflammatory effects. It contains gingerol, a bioactive compound with antioxidant and anti-inflammatory properties. Incorporating fresh ginger into teas, stir-fries, or smoothies can be a flavorful way to benefit from its potential anti-inflammatory effects.

Vitamin D

Vitamin D plays a crucial role in immune system regulation and can influence inflammatory processes. Fatty fish, fortified dairy products, and exposure to sunlight are natural sources of vitamin D. Ensuring an adequate intake of this vitamin may contribute to maintaining a balanced immune response and reducing inflammation.

Fiber

Whole grains, fruits, and vegetables are excellent sources of dietary fiber. Consuming an adequate amount of fiber supports gut health, which is closely linked to inflammation. A healthy gut microbiome can help regulate the immune system and reduce inflammation. Choose whole grains, legumes, and a variety of fruits and vegetables to increase your fiber intake.

Probiotics

Fermented foods like yogurt, kefir, sauerkraut, and kimchi contain probiotics, which are beneficial bacteria that support a healthy gut microbiome. A balanced gut microbiome is associated with reduced inflammation and improved immune function.

Green Tea

Green tea is rich in polyphenols, particularly catechins, which have potent antioxidant and anti-inflammatory properties. Regular consumption of green tea may contribute to reducing inflammation and promoting overall health.

In conclusion, adopting a diet rich in omega-3 fatty acids, antioxidants, turmeric, ginger, vitamin D, fiber, probiotics, and green tea can be instrumental in fighting inflammation. Embracing a variety of nutrient-dense foods and maintaining a balanced lifestyle can have a positive impact on overall health and well-being, helping to keep inflammation at bay. Always consult with a healthcare professional before making significant changes to your diet, especially if you have existing health conditions.

Chapter 5.

Meal Planning and Preparing for Success

In the realm of health and wellness, the concept of anti-inflammatory meal planning has gained significant attention for its potential impact on overall well-being. Chronic inflammation has been linked to various health issues, including heart disease, arthritis, and even certain cancers. Adopting an anti-inflammatory diet involves incorporating foods that are believed to reduce inflammation in the body while excluding those that may contribute to it.

Understanding the Basics of Anti-Inflammatory Diets:

An anti-inflammatory diet is centered around whole, nutrient-dense foods that are rich in antioxidants and anti-inflammatory properties. Key components often include fruits, vegetables, whole grains, lean proteins, and healthy fats. These foods are thought to counteract inflammation by neutralizing free radicals and promoting a balanced immune response.

Meal Planning Strategies:

1. Colorful Plate Approach: Aim to include a variety of colorful fruits and vegetables in every meal. Different hues often signify diverse nutrient profiles, offering a broad range of anti-inflammatory compounds.

2. Omega-3 Fatty Acids: Incorporate sources of omega-3 fatty acids, such as fatty fish (salmon, mackerel, sardines), chia seeds, and flaxseeds.

These essential fats have been shown to have anti-inflammatory effects.

3. Herbs and Spices: Enhance flavor and health benefits by using herbs and spices like turmeric, ginger, garlic, and cinnamon. These ingredients contain natural compounds that possess anti-inflammatory properties.

4. Whole Grains: Opt for whole grains like quinoa, brown rice, and oats instead of refined grains. Whole grains provide fiber and essential

nutrients that support a healthy gut, contributing to overall well-being.

5. Lean Proteins: Choose lean protein sources such as poultry, tofu, legumes, and nuts. These options provide protein without the potential inflammatory effects often associated with processed meats.

Meal Preparation Tips:

1. Batch Cooking: Prepare larger quantities of anti-inflammatory meals and store them in portion-sized containers. This simplifies subsequent meal choices, reducing

the likelihood of opting for less nutritious options.

2. Prep Ahead: Wash, chop, and portion fruits and vegetables in advance. Having these ready-to-go ingredients encourages the inclusion of fresh produce in daily meals.

3. Marinating with Healthy Oils: Use olive oil, known for its anti-inflammatory properties, in marinades for meats or vegetables. The marinating process not only adds flavor but also enhances the

nutritional value of the dish.

4. Experiment with Flavorful Broths: Create homemade broths using ingredients like turmeric, ginger, and garlic. These not only add depth to soups and stews but also provide an additional anti-inflammatory boost.

5. Mindful Eating: Cultivate mindful eating habits by savoring each bite and paying attention to hunger and fullness cues. This approach fosters a healthier relationship with food and can contribute to overall well-

being.

Anti-inflammatory meal planning is not just about what you eat but also how you prepare and consume your meals. By incorporating a variety of nutrient-dense foods and adopting thoughtful preparation practices, you can take proactive steps toward promoting a healthier, more balanced lifestyle that supports inflammation reduction and overall wellness. Remember, small changes in meal planning and preparation can have a lasting impact on your health in the long run.

Chapter 6.

Breakfast Recipes

You may have heard debates about breakfast being the most crucial meal of the day, but these delectable breakfast suggestions aim to kickstart your day with ample energy. Packed with flavors, ranging from savory to sweet, each recipe incorporates anti-inflammatory ingredients known to alleviate symptoms such as brain fog, stiff joints, and digestive issues. Featuring fresh fruits, protein-rich eggs, and leafy greens, these breakfast options are designed to combat inflammation. Notable recipes include Beans on Toast and Berry-Orange Chia Pudding, offering a tasty way to tackle inflammation symptoms throughout the day.

1. Mango-Almond Smoothie Bowl

Ensure the thickness, creaminess, and frostiness of this nutritious smoothie bowl by opting for frozen fruits instead of fresh in this Mango-Almond Smoothie Bowl recipe.

2. Beans on toast

Elevate the classic U.K. beans on toast by incorporating mushrooms for added texture and selenium, along with multigrain bread and chili powder for anti-inflammatory benefits. Top it off with a scrambled or fried egg.

3. Breakfast Salad with Egg & Salsa Verde Vinaigrette

Embrace the unconventional with a Breakfast Salad featuring a generous three cups of vegetables to kickstart your day, complete with a zesty Salsa Verde Vinaigrette.

4. Feta, Egg & Olive Pita

Grab a quick, protein- and fiber-packed breakfast on the go with the Feta, Egg & Olive Pita, assembled in a whole-grain pita for a flavorful start to your day.

5. Chickpea & Kale Toast

Savor a savory bite with the Chickpea & Kale Toast, combining chickpeas, kale, and feta on a slice of healthy toast.

6. Spinach, Peanut Butter & Banana Smoothie

Elevate the classic Peanut Butter & Banana combo with probiotic-rich kefir and mild-flavored spinach in this Spinach, Peanut Butter & Banana Smoothie.

7. Berry-Orange Chia Pudding

Prepare a Berry-Orange Chia Pudding before bedtime for a delightful morning treat, combining chia seeds, coconut milk, berries, and orange juice for a healthy grab-and-go breakfast.

8. Mediterranean flavors with Egg Sandwiches

Indulge in Mediterranean flavors with Egg Sandwiches featuring rosemary, tomato, and feta, creating hearty breakfast sandwiches.

9. Egg in a Hole

Enjoy a colorful and healthy twist on the classic "Egg in a Hole" with bell pepper rings standing in for bread and topped with avocado salsa.

10. Swiss-inspired Bircher Muesli

Dive into the refreshing Swiss-inspired Bircher Muesli, featuring fresh apple, lemon juice, nuts, chia seeds, and fresh berries for a flavorful and nutritious start.

11. Skillet Eggs

Experience a burst of flavor with Skillet Eggs cooked in a mixture of spinach, herbs, and tomatillos, garnished with harissa and perfect for dipping whole-grain country bread.

12. Berry-Almond Smoothie Bowl

Tantalize your taste buds with the Berry-Almond Smoothie Bowl, featuring a creamy texture and the goodness of frozen banana.

13. & Black Bean Hash for a fabulous one-pot meal on busy nights.

14. Pistachio & Peach Toast

Transform leftover ricotta into a delightful Pistachio & Peach Toast, ready in just 5 minutes for a swift breakfast.

15. Spinach & Feta Quiche

Enjoy a gluten-free version of Spinach & Feta Quiche with a Sweet Potato Crust, featuring thinly sliced rounds of sweet potatoes for a scalloped shell.

16. Spring Green Frittata

Whip up a quick and versatile Spring Green Frittata with green spring vegetables, tomatoes, and parmesan cheese in just 25 minutes.

17. Breakfast Naan Pizza

Add a tasty spin to your morning eggs with a Breakfast Naan Pizza, creating an easy individual pizza on a prepared naan.

18. Raspberry-Peach-Mango Smoothie Bowl

Dive into the smoothie-bowl craze with a Raspberry-Peach-Mango Smoothie Bowl, customizable with your favorite fruits, nuts, and seeds.

19. West Coast Avocado Toast

Try the West Coast Avocado Toast with hummus, sprouts, and avocado on sprouted whole-wheat bread for a healthy vegan lunch.

20. Pineapple Spinach Smoothie

Experience the tropical delight of a Pineapple Spinach Smoothie, using juice for sweetness and small, shelf-stable cans for convenience.

21. Spinach & Feta Strata

Delight in the make-ahead convenience of the Spinach & Feta Strata, a breakfast casserole with a flavorful egg mixture soaked into the bread.

22. Overnight Matcha Oats

Wake up to a nutritious breakfast with Overnight Matcha Oats topped with blueberries and raspberries for a meal-prep-friendly option.

23. Spinach & Egg Sweet Potato

Toast

Opt for a gluten-free alternative with Spinach & Egg Sweet Potato Toast, topped with spinach, egg, and hot sauce for a delicious variation of eggs Benedict.

24. Cherry-Spinach Smoothie

Boost your intake of anti-inflammatory foods with the Cherry-Spinach Smoothie, featuring kefir, cherries, avocado, almond butter, chia seeds, and spinach.

25. Two-Ingredient Banana

Pancakes

Enjoy a quick and healthy breakfast with Two-Ingredient Banana Pancakes made with eggs and banana, served with maple syrup and yogurt or ricotta cheese.

26. Avocado Toast with Burrata

Indulge in a decadent Avocado Toast with Burrata, taking this breakfast classic to the next level.

27. Spinach & Cheese Breakfast Skillet

Lower hunger hormones with the

700-calorie Spinach & Cheese Breakfast Skillet, perfect for an early, substantial meal.

28. Pineapple Morning Glory Muffins

Delight in gloriously fruit-packed Pineapple Morning Glory Muffins with less sugar, thanks to grated pineapple incorporated into the batter.

29. Baby Kale Breakfast Salad

Start your day right with a Baby Kale Breakfast Salad featuring quinoa and strawberries, incorporating fruit, whole grains, and greens.

30. Acai Bowl

Treat yourself to a delicious Acai Bowl any day of the week, balancing the tartness of acai with banana, coconut water, and mixed berries, and customize toppings to your liking.

Chapter 7

Lunch Recipes

1. Grilled Salmon Salad: Fresh salmon with mixed greens, cherry tomatoes, and a lemon vinaigrette.

2. Quinoa and Vegetable Bowl: Quinoa topped with colorful bell peppers, cucumbers, and a light olive oil dressing.

3. Turmeric Chickpea Wrap: Whole-grain wrap filled with chickpeas, turmeric, spinach, and tahini.

4. Mango Avocado Salad: Ripe

mango, avocado, and arugula drizzled with balsamic glaze.

5. Cauliflower Rice Stir-Fry: Replace rice with cauliflower rice and stir-fry with colorful vegetables and lean protein.

6. Sweet Potato and Lentil Soup: Hearty soup with sweet potatoes, lentils, and a touch of cumin.

7. Salmon and Asparagus Foil Pack: Baked salmon and asparagus seasoned with herbs in a foil pack.

8. Quinoa Stuffed Bell Peppers: Bell

peppers stuffed with quinoa, black beans, corn, and spices.

9. Greek Yogurt Chicken Salad: Shredded chicken mixed with Greek yogurt, celery, and grapes.

10. Zucchini Noodles with Pesto: Spiralized zucchini noodles tossed with homemade basil pesto.

11. Black Bean and Corn Salad: Black beans, corn, cherry tomatoes, and cilantro with a lime dressing.

12. Mushroom and Spinach Omelette: Whisked eggs folded over

sautéed mushrooms and spinach.

13. Cucumber Avocado Rolls: Sliced cucumber filled with avocado, hummus, and cherry tomatoes.

14. Broccoli and Almond Stir-Fry: Broccoli florets and almonds stir-fried with tofu or chicken.

15. Quinoa Tabbouleh: Quinoa, cucumber, tomatoes, and parsley with a lemon dressing.

16. Turkey and Veggie Lettuce Wraps: Lean ground turkey with a medley of colorful vegetables wrapped in

lettuce.

17. Roasted Vegetable Bowl: Roasted sweet potatoes, Brussels sprouts, and carrots over a bed of quinoa.

18. Lemon Garlic Shrimp Skewers: Grilled shrimp skewers marinated in lemon and garlic.

19. Kale and Berry Smoothie: Blend kale, mixed berries, and almond milk for a refreshing smoothie.

20. Chia Seed Pudding with Berries: Chia seeds soaked in almond milk

topped with fresh berries.

21. Spinach and Feta Stuffed Chicken Breast: Baked chicken breast filled with spinach and feta.

22. Sweet Potato and Chickpea Curry: A warm and comforting curry with sweet potatoes and chickpeas.

23. Cabbage and Carrot Slaw: Shredded cabbage and carrots with a light vinaigrette.

24. Tuna and White Bean Salad: Tuna mixed with white beans, red onion, and a lemony dressing.

25. Roasted Red Pepper Hummus Wrap: Whole-grain wrap filled with hummus, roasted red peppers, and arugula.

26. Eggplant and Tomato Stack: Layers of grilled eggplant, tomato, and mozzarella.

27. Chicken and Vegetable Skewers: Grilled skewers with chicken, bell peppers, and zucchini.

28. Cauliflower and Leek Soup: Creamy soup made with cauliflower, leeks, and vegetable broth.

29. Pesto Zoodle Bowl:Zucchini noodles tossed with pesto, cherry tomatoes, and pine nuts.

30. Salmon and Avocado Sushi Bowl: Deconstructed sushi bowl with salmon, avocado, and brown rice.

Chapter 8

Dinner Recipes

1. Grilled Salmon with Turmeric and Ginger: Packed with omega-3s and anti-inflammatory spices.

2. Quinoa Salad with Mixed Vegetables: Quinoa provides protein, while veggies offer anti-inflammatory benefits.

3. Chicken Stir-Fry with Broccoli and Bell Peppers: Lean protein and colorful veggies make a nutritious, inflammation-fighting dish.

4. Lentil Soup: Rich in fiber and plant -based protein, lentils contribute to reducing inflammation.

5. Baked Sweet Potato with Chickpea Chili: Sweet potatoes and chickpeas combine for a tasty anti-inflammatory meal.

6. Spinach and Mushroom Omelette: Eggs, spinach, and mushrooms offer a nutrient-dense, inflammation-reducing option.

7. Zucchini Noodles with Pesto and Cherry Tomatoes: A low-carb, veggie -packed alternative with the anti-

inflammatory benefits of basil.

8. Turkey and Vegetable Skewers: Lean turkey and a variety of colorful vegetables create a satisfying, anti-inflammatory dinner.

9. Quinoa Stuffed Bell Peppers: Quinoa provides a protein boost, while bell peppers offer anti-inflammatory properties.

10. Grilled Chicken Salad with Avocado: A refreshing salad with lean protein and healthy fats to combat inflammation.

11. Roasted Brussels Sprouts with Walnuts: Brussels sprouts and walnuts are both known for their anti-inflammatory properties.

12. Shrimp and Broccoli Stir-Fry: Shrimp and broccoli team up for a quick, anti-inflammatory dinner option.

13. Mediterranean Chickpea Salad: A flavorful blend of chickpeas, veggies, and olive oil for an anti-inflammatory boost.

14. Baked Cod with Lemon and Herbs: Cod is a lean fish that pairs

well with anti-inflammatory ingredients like lemon and herbs.

15. Cauliflower Fried Rice with Tofu: A low-carb alternative to traditional fried rice with tofu providing plant-based protein.

16. Turkey and Vegetable Soup: A hearty soup with lean turkey and an assortment of veggies for anti-inflammatory benefits.

17. Salmon and Asparagus Foil Packets: A simple and flavorful way to prepare salmon and asparagus, both rich in anti-inflammatory

nutrients.

18. Quinoa and Black Bean Bowl: A protein-packed bowl with quinoa and black beans to support an anti-inflammatory diet.

19. Chicken and Vegetable Curry: Turmeric and other spices in curry contribute to its anti-inflammatory properties.

20. Roasted Eggplant and Tomato Salad: A colorful salad with eggplant and tomatoes, both known for their anti-inflammatory effects.

21. Stir-Fried Tofu with Bok Choy: Tofu and bok choy create a satisfying and anti-inflammatory stir-fry.

22. Baked Chicken with Lemon and Rosemary: Lean chicken paired with anti-inflammatory herbs for a simple yet flavorful dish.

23. Lentil and Vegetable Stir-Fry: Lentils add a protein boost to this veggie-packed stir-fry with anti-inflammatory potential.

24. Cabbage and Carrot Slaw with Ginger Dressing: A crunchy slaw with

a ginger dressing for added anti-inflammatory benefits.

25. Turkey and Spinach Meatballs: Lean turkey and spinach make a tasty and anti-inflammatory meatball option.

26. Grilled Swordfish with Mango Salsa: Swordfish and mango combine for a delicious dish with anti-inflammatory properties.

27. Chickpea and Spinach Stew: A hearty stew with chickpeas and spinach, both contributing to an anti -inflammatory diet.

28. Quinoa and Kale Stuffed Acorn Squash: A nutrient-dense and anti-inflammatory option for a satisfying dinner.

29. Lemon Garlic Shrimp Skewers: Shrimp, lemon, and garlic create a flavorful, anti-inflammatory skewer option.

30. Cucumber and Avocado Salad: A refreshing salad with cucumber and avocado, both known for their anti-inflammatory benefits.

Chapter 9.

Snack and Dessert Recipes

1. Turmeric Roasted Chickpeas:

A crunchy, flavorful snack with the anti-inflammatory benefits of turmeric.

2. Berry Medley Smoothie Bowl:

Packed with antioxidants from berries, this smoothie bowl is not only delicious but also anti-inflammatory.

3. Dark Chocolate Almond Clusters:

Dark chocolate contains anti-inflammatory properties, and paired with almonds, it makes a satisfying treat.

4. Cucumber Avocado Salsa:

A refreshing and inflammation-fighting salsa that pairs well with whole-grain crackers or veggie sticks.

5. Greek Yogurt Parfait with Walnuts and Honey:

Probiotics in Greek yogurt combined with walnuts and honey create a tasty, anti-inflammatory parfait.

6. Baked Sweet Potato Chips:

Thinly sliced sweet potatoes baked to perfection for a crispy, nutrient-rich snack.

7. Chia Seed Pudding with Mango:

Chia seeds are loaded with omega-3 fatty acids, and paired with mango, this pudding is a delicious anti-inflammatory option.

8. Spinach and Artichoke Stuffed Mushrooms:

Mushrooms and spinach are both known for their anti-inflammatory properties, making these stuffed mushrooms a healthy choice.

9. Roasted Red Pepper Hummus with Veggie Sticks:

Hummus, made from chickpeas and infused with red pepper, is a flavorful and anti-inflammatory dip.

10. Coconut Blueberry Energy Bites:

A no-bake snack combining coconut, blueberries, and oats for a tasty anti-inflammatory treat.

11. Mango Turmeric Smoothie:

Blend mango, turmeric, and ginger

for a refreshing, inflammation-fighting smoothie.

12. Quinoa Salad with Mixed Veggies:

A hearty salad with quinoa, loaded with colorful vegetables, providing anti-inflammatory benefits.

13. Edamame Guacamole:

Guacamole gets an anti-inflammatory boost with the addition of protein-packed edamame.

14. Baked Apples with Cinnamon:

Apples contain antioxidants, and

when baked with cinnamon, it becomes a comforting and anti-inflammatory dessert.

15. Broccoli and Cheese Bites:

Broccoli's anti-inflammatory properties shine in these cheesy, bite-sized snacks.

16. Pomegranate Yogurt Bark:

Combine the goodness of pomegranate seeds with yogurt for a frozen, anti-inflammatory dessert.

17. Almond Butter Stuffed Dates:

A simple yet satisfying treat that

combines the natural sweetness of dates with the richness of almond butter.

18. Kale Chips:

 Crispy kale chips seasoned with anti -inflammatory spices like garlic and turmeric.

19. Baked Salmon Bites:

 Salmon is rich in omega-3 fatty acids, making these baked bites both delicious and anti- inflammatory.

20. Mixed Berry Sorbet:

A refreshing sorbet made with mixed berries, offering a sweet way to combat inflammation.

21. Avocado Chocolate Mousse:

Creamy chocolate mousse made with the anti-inflammatory goodness of avocados.

22. Spiced Nuts Mix:

Roasted nuts with a blend of anti-inflammatory spices like cinnamon, turmeric, and cayenne pepper.

23. Papaya Lime Sorbet:

Papaya's enzymes combined with

lime create a tropical and anti-inflammatory dessert.

24. Olive Tapenade with Whole Grain Toast:

Olives contain compounds with anti-inflammatory properties, perfect for a flavorful tapenade.

25. Apricot and Almond Energy Balls:

A quick and easy snack featuring apricots and almonds, known for their anti-inflammatory benefits.

26. Minty Watermelon Salad:

Watermelon paired with mint

creates a hydrating, anti-inflammatory snack.

27. Roasted Beet Chips:

Thinly sliced beets roasted to perfection for a vibrant and nutritious snack.

28. Cacao Nib Almond Butter Cups:

A healthier twist on the classic peanut butter cup, using almond butter and cacao nibs.

29. Green Tea Chia Seed Pudding:

Green tea adds an antioxidant boost to this chia seed pudding, promoting anti-inflammatory effects.

30. Cinnamon Roasted Butternut Squash:

Butternut squash roasted with cinnamon for a sweet and anti-inflammatory side or snack.

Chapter 10.

Anti-Inflammatory Beverages

1. Green Tea:

Stuffed with cancer prevention agents, green tea has anti-inflammatory properties.

2. Turmeric Latte:

Turmeric's dynamic compound, curcumin, is known for its anti-inflammatory impacts.

3. Ginger Tea:

Ginger contains gingerol, which has anti-inflammatory and antioxidant properties.

4. Pineapple Smoothie:

Bromelain in pineapple has anti-inflammatory benefits.

5. Beetroot Juice:

Betalains in beets show anti-inflammatory impacts.

6. Matcha Latte:

Matcha is wealthy in cancer prevention agents that combat aggravation.

7. Brilliant Drain:

Combining turmeric with warm drain gives a relieving anti-inflammatory drink.

8. Blueberry Smoothie:

Blueberries contain anthocyanins with anti-inflammatory properties.

9. Coconut Water:

Hydrating and may offer assistance diminish irritation.

10. Rosehip Tea:

Tall in vitamin C and cancer prevention agents, known for anti-inflammatory impacts.

11. Tart Cherry Juice:

Contains anthocyanins, which have anti-inflammatory and antioxidant impacts.

12. Lemon Water:

Vitamin C in lemons can offer assistance combat aggravation.

13. Cucumber Mint Imbued Water:

Hydrating with anti-inflammatory properties.

14. Chamomile Tea:

Known for its calming and anti-inflammatory impacts.

15. Aloe Vera Juice:

May offer assistance diminish irritation and advance mending.

16. Carrot Ginger Juice:

Carrots and ginger both have anti-inflammatory properties.

17. Pomegranate Juice:

Stuffed with cancer prevention agents that battle aggravation.

18. Dandelion Tea:

May have anti-inflammatory and

detoxifying impacts.

19. Lavender Lemonade:

Lavender may have calming and anti
-inflammatory benefits.

20. Hibiscus Tea:

Wealthy in cancer prevention agents,
hibiscus has anti-inflammatory
properties.

21. Watermelon Juice:

Contains lycopene, which has anti-
inflammatory impacts.

22. Mint Tea:

Menthol in mint has anti-inflammatory and relieving properties.

23. Celery Juice:

May have anti-inflammatory benefits and back assimilation.

24. Elderberry Syrup:

Contains cancer prevention agents that will offer assistance decrease aggravation.

25. Cinnamon Coffee:

Cinnamon has anti-inflammatory and antioxidant properties.

26. Spinach and Kale Smoothie:

Verdant greens are wealthy in anti-inflammatory compounds.

27. Orange Carrot Turmeric Juice:

A combination of anti-inflammatory fixings.

28. Kiwi and Strawberry Implanted Water:

Both natural products have anti-inflammatory properties.

29. Vex Tea:

Vex has anti-inflammatory and

antioxidant impacts.

30. Avocado Smoothie:

Avocado's monounsaturated fats may have anti-inflammatory benefits.

Chapter 11.

Adapted Recipes for Specific Dietary Needs

In our differing world, people frequently explore through different dietary prerequisites due to wellbeing conditions, individual choices, or social inclinations. Making dinners that cater to particular dietary needs can be both a challenge and a inventive opportunity. In this chapter, we'll investigate adjusted formulas for different dietary contemplations, advertising options and substitutions to oblige a wide run of dietary prerequisites.

1. Gluten-Free Delights

For those with gluten affectability or celiac illness, getting a charge out of scrumptious dinners without compromising taste is pivotal. Testing with elective flours such as almond, coconut, or chickpea flour can change conventional formulas. Attempt a gluten-free pizza outside with a mix of rice and custard flour for a firm, fulfilling result.

2. Low-Carb Ponders

People taking after a low-carb way of life regularly look for innovative ways to supplant high-carb fixings. Cauliflower, zucchini, and spaghetti squash make fabulous substitutes for rice and pasta. Jump into the world of spiralized vegetables to form fulfilling noodle choices, opening the entryway to a plenty of low-carb culinary experiences.

3. Dairy-Free Liberalities

For those who are lactose narrow minded or take after a dairy-free eat less, finding wealthy and rich options is key. Coconut drain, almond drain, and cashew cream can be utilized in put of conventional dairy items in formulas. Investigate the craftsmanship of making dairy-free ice creams utilizing solidified bananas or coconut drain for a luscious treat.

4. Vegan and Vegetarian Wonders

Vegan and veggie lover diets are picking up notoriety, and adjusting formulas to prohibit creature items opens up a world of plant-based conceivable outcomes. Grasp the flexibility of tofu, tempeh, and vegetables as protein sources. Make dynamic and flavorful dishes with a rainbow of vegetables, displaying the magnificence and differences of plant-based food.

5. Nut-Free Options

Exploring a nut-free way of life requires imagination to preserve both flavor and surface in formulas. Sunflower seeds, pumpkin seeds, and oats can be substituted for nuts in granolas and vitality bars. Nut-free pesto made with basil, spinach, or arugula gives a new bend to pasta dishes, guaranteeing a secure and delicious encounter for those with nut hypersensitivities.

6. Sugar-Free Sweetness

Decreasing or dispensing with refined sugar from formulas doesn't cruel relinquishing sweetness. Investigate normal sweeteners like maple syrup, nectar, or agave nectar. Date glue and squashed bananas include characteristic sweetness to prepared merchandise, giving a more beneficial elective whereas keeping up the required flavor profile.

7. Heart-Healthy Choices

For those centered on heart wellbeing, joining omega-3-rich nourishments and incline proteins is fundamental. Salmon, chia seeds, and flaxseeds can be coordinates into suppers to bolster cardiovascular well-being. Explore with herbs and flavors to improve flavor without depending on over the top salt or immersed fats.

In conclusion, adjusting formulas to

meet particular dietary needs permits for a broadened culinary involvement, cultivating inclusivity within the world of gastronomy. Whether it's gluten-free, low-carb, dairy-free, vegan, nut-free, sugar-free, or heart-healthy, embracing differing qualities in our cooking not as it were addresses person needs but too celebrates the wealthy embroidered artwork of tastes and inclinations that make up our worldwide community. So, wear your smock, set out on a culinary travel, and savor the bliss of creating meals that cater to everyone's interesting dietary necessities.

Chapter 12

Tips for Sustaining an Anti-Inflammatory Lifestyle

Keeping up an anti-inflammatory way of life is vital for generally wellbeing and well-being. Inveterate irritation has been connected to different wellbeing issues, counting heart illness, diabetes, and immune system disarranges. Embracing propensities that advance an anti-inflammatory environment in your body can contribute to long-term wellbeing benefits. Here are a few tips to assist you maintain an anti-inflammatory way of life:

1. Nutrient-Rich Count calories:

Center on a slim down wealthy in natural products, vegetables, entire grains, and incline proteins. These nourishments are stacked with cancer prevention agents and phytochemicals that combat irritation.

-Join omega-3 greasy acids found in greasy angle, flaxseeds, and walnuts. These fats have anti-inflammatory properties.

2. Constrain Handled Nourishments:

Decrease your admissions of handled and refined nourishments, as they regularly contain trans fats, sugar, and manufactured added substances that can contribute to aggravation.

3. Hydration is Key:

Remain enough hydrated by drinking bounty of water all through the day. Legitimate hydration makes a difference flush out poisons and bolsters different real capacities that play a part in diminishing aggravation.

4. Oversee Stretch:

Persistent stretch can trigger aggravation. Join stress-management procedures such as reflection, profound breathing, yoga, or mindfulness hones into your every day schedule.

5. Satisfactory Rest:

Guarantee you get adequate, quality rest each night. Need of rest can contribute to inflammation and compromise your safe framework.

6. Customary Work out:

Lock in in customary physical movement. Work out has anti-inflammatory impacts and makes a difference keep up a sound weight, lessening the chance of inflammation-related conditions.

7. Adjusted Intestine Wellbeing:

Expend probiotic-rich nourishments like yogurt, kefir, and aged vegetables to advance a solid intestine microbiome. A adjusted intestine contributes to a lower chance of irritation.

8. Herbs and Flavors:

Consolidate anti-inflammatory herbs and flavors such as turmeric, ginger, garlic, and cinnamon into your dinners. These fixings contain compounds that can offer assistance combat aggravation.

9. Restrain Liquor and Tobacco:

Over the top liquor utilization and smoking can contribute to aggravation. Restrain or maintain a strategic distance from these substances to back an anti-inflammatory way of life.

10. Standard Wellbeing Check-ups:

Plan standard check-ups together with your healthcare supplier to screen your generally wellbeing. Recognizing and tending to potential wellbeing issues early can avoid inflammation-related complications.

11. Keep up a Sound Weight:

Overabundance body weight, particularly visceral fat, is related with irritation. Receiving a adjusted slim down and standard work out can offer assistance accomplish and keep up a solid weight.

12. Anti-Inflammatory Supplements:

Counsel with a healthcare proficient approximately consolidating anti-inflammatory supplements such as angle oil, curcumin, and quercetin into your schedule.

Remember that receiving an anti-inflammatory way of life may be a all encompassing approach that includes numerous angles of your day by day schedule. Consistency and commitment to these propensities can contribute to a more beneficial, inflammation-resistant body over time. Continuously counsel with healthcare experts for personalized exhortation based on your person wellbeing needs and conditions.

Conclusion.

In conclusion, this anti-inflammatory diet cookbook speaks to a essential asset within the domain of all encompassing wellbeing and nourishment. Through a fastidious mix of culinary imagination and evidence-based wholesome intelligence, it rises above the ordinary boundaries of cookbooks, developing as a comprehensive direct to developing well-being from inside.

The culinary travel set out upon within these pages isn't simply a collection of recipes but a transformative encounter established within the standards of anti-inflammatory eating. By honestly curating fixings known for their anti-inflammatory properties, the cookbook offers a different and agreeable range of dishes that amplify past the insignificant fulfillment of taste buds. It gets to be a catalyst for a way of life move, empowering people to produce a more profound association between the nourishment they devour and the affect it has on their generally wellbeing.

What sets this cookbook separated is its immovable commitment to wedding gastronomic charm with dietary importance. Each formula serves as a culinary experience, fastidiously outlined to not as it were tantalize the faculties but moreover contribute to the diminishment of aggravation inside the body. From vibrant salads to generous fundamental courses and liberal sweets, each dish may be a confirmation to the conviction that nutritious eating require not give up flavor.

Besides, the consideration of nitty gritty dietary information and instructive bits of knowledge hoists this cookbook past the domain of simple formulas. It gets to be a trusted companion for those on a travel towards wellness, engaging them with information almost the science behind anti-inflammatory eating. Perusers are not fair inactive beneficiaries of formulas; they are dynamic participants in an educated and careful approach to their dietary choices.

As the peruser navigates through the ultimate pages, they rise not as it were with a wealthy collection of culinary motivations but too with a recharged understanding of the significant affect their dietary choices can have on their by and large wellbeing. The anti-inflammatory count calories ceases to be a prohibitive set of rules; it changes into a freeing and feasible way of life, cultivating long-term well-being.

In pith, this anti-inflammatory eat less cookbook is more than a compilation of recipes; it could be a celebration of wellbeing, a combination of gastronomy and sustenance that rises above the boundaries of conventional cookbooks. It stands as a confirmation to the thought that eating for wellness can be both delightful and transformative, advertising a guide for those looking for to savor the travel towards a dynamic and inflammation-free life.

www.ingramcontent.com/pod-product-compliance
Lightning Source LLC
Chambersburg PA
CBHW070758260726
48660CB00005B/1677